CONTENTS DISCOVER THE SECRETS OF AWAKENED WOMEN!

When is the moment of awakening coming?

We become awakened women when we clearly recognize our values and live our days with higher spiritual awareness.

We feed our relationships, members of our family, build our businesses, do our job from this consciousness.

I think that awakening does not mean raising awareness of our current roles, but recognizing our brilliant being, and we are watching the world with the heart of this pure wonderful being.

The turning point is the moment when Kore wakes up her consciousness and becomes Persephone, who goes beyond the shadows of the girl to become the goddess of the shadows.

I really like Persephone's story. It is a road which we also walk on as women.

We often meet our shadows - finances, family, partners, religious community, social expectations, sickness, dislike, worthlessness, rape, shame, domestic violence - which burden our shoulders with heavy weights.

When faced with them, (we consciously find the shadows that make us feel incomplete and we are unable to unfold) we face the first phase of awakening.

This is the alarm, which does not guarantee awakening.

You can choose freely. You can ask for your power or leave your fort, which helps to make changes.

You can say that you know it's not okay, but you cannot change it by saying that it was enough.Pick yourself up and find a solution.It is always your decision, but I'm sure that If you read this magazine, you will be ready to get out of your shadow into light and show your magical feminine glow!

THERESIA VALOCZY

www.consciouscreatorspublishing.com

THE AWAKENED FEMININE SOUL

By Joanne Cruise

What dwells in the heart of an awakened woman?
Are we the wild and free goddess of nature?
Maybe, the nourishing, giver of life?
Or, the mysterious and wise soul of the spiritual seeker?

When we, as women, open our hearts to walk the path of
our awakened spirit, all the possibilities that life offers
us intensifies.
The sacred breath of the Divine feminine fire burns
bright within the passion of our creative expression.
Our voices unite and bring forth the utterings of our
ancestors.
The way of the wild woman is free to roam the land.
Scattering the seeds of love to bloom into the next
generations.
We reveal the worlds womb, from which all life springs
forth. The deep well of boundless love and creation, of
which woman is life's keeper.

As our heart's stir to the whisperings of the truth of who
we are: -
We release our 'egoic' based desires.
We surrender to the Universal flow of life.
We embrace our sacred soul power.

We embody the truth of our authentic nature.
We collaborate, celebrate and combine forces.

We are the river of life flowing through the veins of our
Mother Earth.
We are the ebb and flow of the tides.
We are the beating heart of Gaia.
We feel love like the depths of the oceans.
We rise together to meet the stars and moon and sun.

We laugh and cry and dance and sing.
We are the untameable hearts, the unapologetically
liberated souls.
We are the descendants of wise women, old crones and
shamans of old.
We are the fighters of truth and justice, the healers and
lovers.
We are the bringers of life, creating bonds of infinite,
unconditional love.

We are the women with awakened hearts.
We stand as one - united by love
We celebrate our inspired gifts, from above
When women embrace their love for all
The world shines brighter, like never before.

We are the nurturers, protectors and bearers of life

The sister, the mother, the daughter, the wife
We share wisdom and knowledge passed down through the years
We are the vessels of the sacred mysteries of women's joys and tears.

We each hold the banner of love in our heart,
The strength of which can never be broken apart
And when others look back and celebrate our life and light
They'll feel in their hearts our awakened love for them shine bright

About Joanne

Joanne Cruise - BA (Hons) IIHHT.

Author & Co-Founder of Holistic Angels® & Joanne Cruise the Word Angel.

Joanne supports women to; realise their full and creative expression, embrace a holistic lifestyle & to awaken their sacred feminine soul. Joanne's passionate about helping women fulfil their potential through the mind, body & spirit connection. For over twenty years she has facilitated hundreds of women on their journeys of self-discovery & empowerment.

Find out more and connect with Joanne

www.joannecruise.co.uk
www.facebook.com/jocruise777
www.twitter.com/jo_crui
www.Instagram.com/joanne_cruise

THE SEXUALLY AWAKENING WOMAN

By Natasha Botkin

In my opinion the definition of an awakened woman is a woman who is willing to go into every depth of her soul and can meet this in a manner that is the Spiritual, Physical, Emotional and Mental embodiment of the Soul. A higher calling into who she is rather that what she has been taught or sought to believe. She can move beyond the boundaries that once bound her to a false sense. She has unleashed, unraveled and let go of the old to make way for the new. This may not be an easy road to travel per say. Rather it is about going into those dark depths of your soul and meeting you. You may need to move from the dark into the light and then again into the brink of darkness which casts your illumination into the path of your   lightness.

Once upon a time I fell in love with the adage and notions of true love, first kiss and all that fun filled ideas that little girls are raised to believe. However, on my path, I found that to be quite untrue and sequestered a very dark depth into the cavity of my small self (ego). Which created a huge nuisance for me and the declaration, "What man would possibly want a powerful woman?" Therefore, I went down a path of internal condemnation: To receive love, I would have to weaken myself. This is false and is the essence of the smaller self (ego) coming forth. When I let go of that declared vow, I found myself with what could be called true love's form.

There is a path of an awakened woman that is not always spoken about; an awakened woman needs a love partner who is going to challenge her, but also be alright when this happens. Hence what was coming forth for me is: "can I find a powerful enough partner who can help challenge me in those kinds of ways." This isn't to say that it is all bad; yet, there are times when we are all afraid. How do you accept fear? For me, there have been moments where fear did not phase me. Unfortunately, there have been fears moments where I felt the need to run and hide. For me it is about accepting me at my most authentic truth and to be gentle with myself. This is about the journey rather than the destination. It is not about who is winning or who has more trophies.

This is the exploration and discovery of who I am; the absolute true authenticity of your soul. It is about a woman loving herself and granting her mate to love all of her. This is allowing each other to be beautiful beings even in the darkest moments. So, love for me as an awakened woman is powerful, caring, kind, sexual and loving. A free, kindred spirit who is willing to tap into her darker depths while exploring her light. Conceding with your partner brings forth your sexual vibrancy. By permitting this individual to meet you in those dark or light moments, you are accepting your sexual being on a whole other level. You are going into crevasses that may not have ever been reached before; thus, allowing your sexual powers, energies and vibrancy to emerge. There are moments that will be spectacular. They will feel free and exhilarating. There may be moments when challenges will arise. How will you accept and allow yourself to explore your inner depths? Are you also willing to allow your partner to explore these beautiful inner depths? This can create a deep Divine pulsing essence more than ever before and bring forth a power to be unleashed to enjoy.

Part of my fear with my BeLoved was what would he see in those depths. Which led to, I have no idea what or even how to experience those deep sexual encounters between the two of us. However, by stepping away from control and to begin allowing the beautiful essence of a man and a woman making love creates an energy vibrancy like no other. As the depth of my soul arises, so does he. When I was saying that men are afraid of a powerful woman; it is not necessarily her looks or intelligence; this is the much deeper depth of her sexual being. She is being brought forth in the most divinely radiant manner. This awakens the beautiful sexual vitality upon which we ladies are. I was asking for my mate to accept all of me in my power, and I was also asking for a mate to recognizes his own power and that he   too,   is   powerful.

There is an even deeper awakening that occurs as two share, explore and dive into their powers. The unleashing of shame creates an intense spark of deep inner gift. A woman in her own Divine radiant powers is a dynamic creative being. The creative preemptiveness surges and pours out in the most incredible manner. Ladies, go forth and enjoy the sexual awakening of these beautiful vibrant energies. These have been forsaken and put to sleep for far too long. Join me by awakening your woman's sexual being and unleashing the deep depths of your   soul.

About Natasha

Natasha Botkin, Master Teacher & Intuitive Behavioral Energy Healer, is a #1 international bestselling author and Shiny Gold Star Quest creator. She uses healing soul psychology energies when working with youth and adults by releasing patterns & blocks to help them empower themselves.   Connect   with   me

www.magicalblessingshealingcenter.com

AWAKENING TO YOUR SELF

By   Marisa   Ferrera

The following MESSAGE FROM THE LIGHT was channeled through Marisa Ferrera on october 16, 2014

From humble beginnings many men and women have done great things. All it takes is a willingness to stand in Truth and not back down in the face of opposition. There will always be those who will oppose anything that is new, anything that rattles the status quo, for it takes strength and courage to be different, to be YOU.

You are each unique and special and yet you try to be the same in order to fit it and not be noticed. You feel safer and more loved when you experience the acceptance of others and yet oftentimes it is at the expense of rejecting yourself. What you do not realize is that no matter how you show up in your world, there will be those who will love you and those who will reject you so why not be who you are?

The more you live YOUR life and not the life of an imposter, the happier you will be and the more you will experience life as pleasurable rather than as a struggle and full of pain. Your pain is your measuring stick that tells you how close you are to your Truth. The more pain you feel, the further away you are. It's like the game "hot and cold."

As you connect more and more to YOUR TRUTH, you will experience less and less pain and struggle in your life. Let pain be your guide and pay attention to it. Ask your pain what it is trying to tell you and listen. Give thanks for your pain for it has a purpose and that purpose is to lead you back to YOU…to who you really are.

Marisa's Musings

This sounds so simple, and yet I know from personal experience how challenging it can be. I grew up in an environment where I learned it was safer to keep quiet than to ever challenge what my father believed to be true. After leaving home in my late teens to further my education, I discovered that I had no idea who I was. If anyone asked me how I felt about something or what I liked or didn't like, I couldn't answer them.

Recognizing this about myself terrified me. I remember thinking, *"How can I ever love someone or feel someone's love for me if I can't feel anything?"* I suffered a great deal of emotional pain and loneliness. I recognized in my early 20's that unless I got help, I would likely feel this pain and loneliness for the rest of my life.

Not only did I seek counseling and read a number of self help books, I also asked God, my angels and guides to help me. I didn't realize it at that time, but this is when I began the journey of awakening. It was an inward journey that continues to this day as I discover more and more about who I am and what I wish to experience in my life.

I have become an advocate for authentic communication and encourage everyone to speak THEIR TRUTH (from their heart) no matter what others may think. It's not always easy and yet it is so liberating. I have discovered that the more I express myself authentically with others, the safer they feel to express their truth with me.

When I look back and see how far I've come, I feel so grateful and blessed for the joyful and love-filled life I am living today.

About Marisa

Marisa Ferrera
Soul-Centered Relationship Coach
#1 International Best Selling Author of *"Magnify Your Magnificence:*
Your Pathway to the Life & Relationships You Truly Desire"(to get a copy of this book go to: MagnifyYourMagnificence.com*)*

MarisaFerrera.com

AN AWAKENED WOMAN: THE LAST SINGLE GIRL

By Valerie Naidoo

When I think about the men I dated in my 20s, compared to the men I date in my late 30's; I'm glad that I didn't get married back then! Women are dictating the pace of dating and with many prioritizing their careers over personal/social commitments – the white fairy tale wedding is becoming more of an illusion. Having said this; carving out a high profile career and owning the lifestyle versus finding the one and racing against the fertility clock looms largely in the background for many – I am not alone in this.

I am a 4th generation South African Indian; conditioned to act and think British. Due to spending the better part of my twenties and early thirties in the UK and a few other countries, I have learnt to relate to the multi-dimensional first world mind-set. My journey has led me far and beyond; I have awakened to the fact that the higher spirit lives within me and I'm guided by the *Holy Spirit* and being *"the last single girl"* no longer matters.

For women who are well into their thirties and edging into their forties, it's no longer a money issue – you have the option to own your time and lifestyle and most importantly to live a life of purpose. In the past I've experienced a circle of hell in trying to explain my reasons for not opting for an early marriage and how the need to live independently has forever beckoned me. Not marrying early and not having kids – does this mean that I'm unhappy, that I've not reached a desired state and that I'm unhealthy and miserable? We seem to be ruled by certain levels of controversy – many in society still prescribe to these out-dated norms.

I feel that a fear to go against social grains, often leave some individuals punctuated with uncertainty. The femosphere is encouraged to be ambitious, but we should not be overly ambitious, we can be outspoken but not too outspoken, we need to shrink on certain levels – otherwise we will intimidate the opposite sex. Females are often far too harshly judged; for not marrying at an early age, for getting divorced, for marrying men far too older or younger than us or even for not being able to bear children. We live in a society governed by social norms that tend to define thinking patterns and choices. Yet as society on a whole we're missing the big picture – this journey isn't only about marriage, wealth, status and kids but more on the lines of living out your destiny.

Have you ever asked yourself "what is my God given purpose and how am I meant to serve?" Sadly most of the highly educated and super wealthy don't have the answers to these fundamental questions. It is time to get off the conventional path and awaken ourselves from within! As women we need to re-programme to connect with our inner selves and in doing so we will receive the most amounts of gratification and success in all domains. Spending just 30 minutes a day praying, meditating and doing yoga has shifted the energy in my heart from that of fear and stress to immense joy and confidence. These days the moment my eyes opens I feel the joy of God and life immersing from my heart and radiating my being and no matter what the day brings – nothing can rob me off my joy.

I don't think there is ever a right or wrong time to marry and finding *"the one"* should not be dictated at the pace of the media or society. Women; married or single, deserve to have the level of happiness they desire! I celebrate my life because I have found the courage to cross a few big chasms, to stand up to tradition while addressing key social barriers, and I'm comfortable in my skin. I have dared to stand out in my journey personally and professionally by awakening myself to the higher truth. Self awareness has not only raised my thinking and joy but also led to me becoming an awakened woman and today I have indeed become a celebrated *last single girl*.

My coaching fellowship program "Powering up a new Gen of women" does encourage women on building a firm internal foundation that curates self awareness, hence expanding business and career. I would encourage every woman who is able to join me on this program to participate.

About Valerie

ValerieNaidoo is Multiple international best-selling author

Recruiter | Peak Performance coach | Voice & Accent Trainer | Motivational speaker

CEO of WallStreet Coaching Foundation

HOW TO STOP SELLING YOURSELF SHORT

FIVE PRACTICAL TIPS TO TRANSFORM YOUR SELF IMAGE

By Debbra Lupien

You ARE The Equal of Any Other Person

So many women that I speak with have distorted views of themselves. Somewhere along their journey they have been made to feel less than — or inferior —repeatedly.

As a result, many of us are walking around deeply wounded, not understanding our true value. **It's time to stop seeing ourselves as flawed, damaged or unworthy.**

When we have a distorted perception of ourselves, we become predisposed to perceive even off-hand comments as negative — whether they were intended as such or not.

Everything filters through our belief of being less than "others" who we view as smarter, more successful, better looking, etc. We are constantly finding evidence to further prove our unworthiness. It doesn't matter how much we achieve, there's always a feeling of not measuring up.

Life As Viewed Through A Distortion Filter

If that's your truth, then you probably find yourself pooh poohing even the most sincere compliment. Instead of graciously saying "thank you" and feeling good, you begin mentally reviewing all of your shortcomings.

You've developed an extensive list and are intimately familiar with your flaws. You may even cut off the proffered compliment, protesting that it can't be true and then begin explaining in painful detail exactly why. You'll teach that person not to give you another compliment!

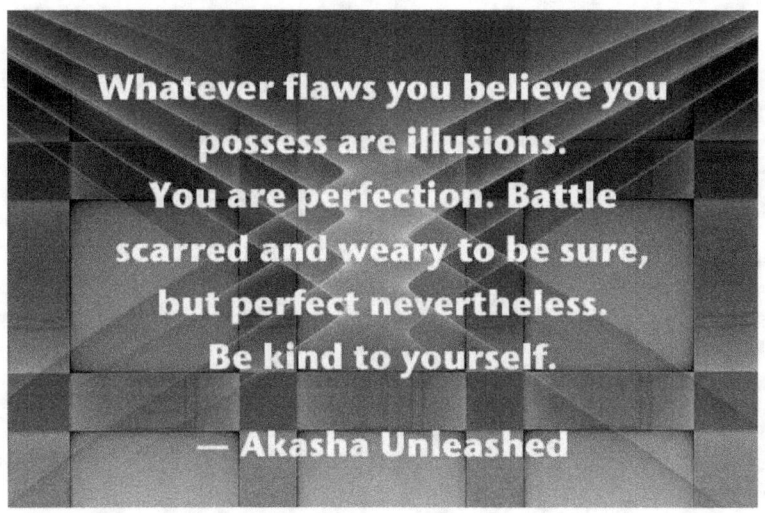

Whatever flaws you believe you possess are illusions.
You are perfection. Battle scarred and weary to be sure, but perfect nevertheless.
Be kind to yourself.

— Akasha Unleashed

Light At The End of The Tunnel

I know all too well what it's like, having gone through my own dark journey for far too long. Fortunately that all changed as a result of discovering truth in the Akashic Records.

Over and over messages came through with a now familiar theme. **You are perfect. Magnificent. The equal of any other. There is nothing wrong with you.**

This message continues to come through regularly. I've discovered there are so many of us who see ourselves as "less than" that it's practically an epidemic. But you know what? Many of those people you look upon as better than you harbor the same insecurities.

So what are we to do about it?

1. See yourself through the eyes of your Akashic Team

Your Akashic Guide team think that you "hung the moon." Truly. They will tell you if you're willing to listen. You are exactly where you're supposed to be based upon the choices you've made — and there's nothing wrong with that. It's all part of your journey. **YOU ARE NOT BROKEN!** You never were.

They want you to understand that they're committed to your success. They always have your back. Isn't it about time that **you** have your back? After all if you can't appreciate yourself how can others? "Love your neighbor as yourself" only works if you first love yourself. Otherwise you have nothing to give your neighbor.

We've gotten it wrong for far too long. It's not selfish to take care of yourself. It's the responsible thing to do. You can't help others if you allow your own "well" to run dry.

Of course it won't happen in the blink of an eye. However, your team wants you to see the big picture and begin the process of self appreciation. Allow your perception to shift and the transformation to begin!

2. It's Time to Recognize Your True Value

Each of us is a masterpiece designed by our genius Creator. How then can we not value ourselves as the magnificent creation that we are? Will you argue with your Creator?

It's time to stop selling yourself short. Time to recognize your true value.

At this time when so many souls are awakening to higher consciousness, Archangel Metatron felt it was important to remind us that part of awakening is recognizing our value.

"It's **time** for the children to awaken. Time to stop walking through life like a zombie, only expressing primal needs. Time to tap into your fifth dimensional, amazing, powerful self and claim your birthright. Time to embrace your power and live life full out with gusto and exquisite joy."

You deserve it and you are worth it!

3. Rewrite The Bad Code

Memories and thoughts we have that uphold beliefs of being "less than" are like bad computer code. They corrupt our self esteem. Just like bad code, they can be eradicated and replaced with "good" code.

You control your reality. **You** control your thoughts. I know it may not seem that way. However, I assure you it's absolutely true (speaking from personal experience). You can absolutely choose to rewrite those memories, replacing them with positive, uplifting ones.

I'm not saying it's easy or instantaneous, but you have the ability to do exactly that.

Let me give you an example:

You are introduced to someone at a party and engage in small talk. Feeling awkward you blurt out something and immediately judge yourself as being socially inept (or whatever script runs in your program). Shortly after, that person excuses themself and walks away.

At this point you probably begin mentally excoriating yourself with all sorts of recriminations about how stupid, clumsy, ugly, etc. you are. An old familiar pattern. *(Frankly so old it should already be extinct!)*

From your new perspective you can choose to write a different script: You had a lovely conversation with a new person. They excused themself (not because of anything you said), but because they had to pee, or make a phone call, or... any number of reasons having nothing to do with you. In fact **you'd be surprised how often it has nothing to do with you**.

In reality you have no idea what they were thinking so why not choose to believe a positive story rather than a negative? That's what free choice is all about. You get to write the story (or code).

What if you retrieved some of those old, painful memories and rewrote them? One by one, rewrite them and focus on your new version until it feels comfortable and true. This really works! Ask me how I know.

4. Choose To Accept And Believe

Resolve that the next time someone pays you a compliment, you will smile and say "thank you." Accept the compliment as sincere and feel good about it.

Practice giving yourself compliments, smiling, and saying "thank you" in the mirror if you need to. The more you accept, the easier it gets.

As you shift into this new perception, you'll feel better and better, until one day you won't even think about it. Your natural response will be to believe and feel pleasure.

5. Install The New Programming Code

Each time an old painful memory comes to mind, replace it with your new version. Dismiss the old story and immediately focus on (and bask in), your wonderful new version.

In the beginning it will be a challenge — after all you've been running those old sound tracks for a very long time. However, with focus and determination you will find (in very short time), it becomes surprisingly easy.

One day you'll notice that you feel so much better about

yourself, all warm and fuzzy. You'll finally comprehend and appreciate the magnificent human being in whose skin you dwell.

About Debbra

Debbra Lupien, The Answer Diva of AkashaUnleashed.com, is an internationally known Akashic Records Expert. She specializes in helping women discover their soul purpose, embrace their magnificence, and unleash their potential. Clarity of purpose is the key to skyrocketing success and happiness. Download your free gift: Well-Being Attunement Meditation today: http://bit.ly/299gSh3

MANIFESTING : WATCH YOUR IMAGINATION

By Reba Linker

Our imaginations lead us on wondrous adventures.

Imagination is key to manifesting everything we desire. Imagination is intrinsic to our creativity – and we are, above all, creative beings.

However, imagination may also lead to great unhappiness.

I'm not speaking of the dangers of imagining horrific things. Many of us already understand how terrible imaginings help produce terrible results in our lives. What we focus on, grows, right?

But I'm not even speaking of that truth.

I'm speaking of how imagining wonderful things may lead to unhappiness – if we are not careful. This is the imagination that always sees the perfect vision, against which we always come up short. This is the imagination that tells us all that we could be, and all that we should have.

1. If we have a potted plant, we imagine that life would be perfect if only we had a small porch or balcony.

2. If we have a balcony, we long for a patch of earth, a little backyard.

3. When we have a backyard, we dwell on what it might be like to live with a view of mountains and wilderness.

4. And on and on…

We do this with our weight, always wishing to be slimmer. We dismiss our achievements, knowing that we are not yet where we wish to be. We long for a different, or upgraded version of home, family and friends. We do this in every area of our lives.

Our beautiful visions of life-as-it-should-be are used by us, against us. They taunt us with the ghost of accomplishments yet to come. They highlight our limitations and lack until we are in danger of losing sight of what we've achieved. Our brilliant visions become weapons in the hands of our inner critic and inner mean girl, a yardstick against which we can never measure up.

As a young dance student, I was a slave to that yardstick for many years. My appreciation of beauty far outstripped my ability to achieve my vision. I was trying to dance from the outside, in. I tried to strike those poses, and hit those lines! I had to learn that it is best to dance from the inside, out. After all, that inner feeling is what made me fall in love with dance in the first place.

Sometimes we have to just let the visions go.

Manifesting our best and happiest life is a delicate balance between the vision of what we desire and gratitude for all that we already have.

Stop longing for perfection, stop chasing the dream. Instead, be happy now.

Be happy now with this imperfect family.

Be happy now with this body just as it is.

Be happy now with these accomplishments to date.
Yes, we have accomplished so much already!

Be happy now even with these challenges that are ours alone to navigate.

Our stories are uniquely wonderful, crazily colorful, all wrong and yet so perfectly right. Embrace the story of

NOW and stop running after the impossible glossy magazine version of what our lives should look like.

Be happy with this day,

with this potted plant,

with this busy life.

The Universe is contained in every blade of grass. All this is already ours.

About Reba

Reba Linker is a bestselling author, life coach, and host of the Youtube interview show, Paint Yourself Into the Picture: http://bit.ly/1rq0fWy.

She is the Founder of a new online community, www.AtoZHealingSpace.com, that celebrates the idea that many different modalities lead to a greater awareness of the self and our partnership with Spirit.

AtoZ Healing Space offers an 'elite' experience in terms of the connection and caring you receive as a member, and in terms of the excellence of what we provide.

NOT elitist is the affordable price.

For less than a cup of coffee a day, you are invited to life-changing workshops and events. Learn more with this sampling of gifts from some of our featured healers: http://www.atozhealingspace.com/free-gift/

KORE'S KIDNAPPING

By Theresia Valoczy

Following the events of our lives in the light, Kore's(Persephone's) kidnapping occurs when we forget our true personality, forget to be.

Behind every negative fact is that many women are related to the life of man.

In all events which lead to loss of self-confidence, low self-esteem blurs the self, more pain acts as a protective envelope by placing our souls in it.

After the abduction pains, fears about our saturated subordinate selves in the shade will settle upon us.

A 42-year-old woman tells the story of this period:

"I was 34 when a man confronted me in the street and took my wallet. I was alone, there was no one nearby. I was so scared that I could barely stand. Feeling weak blocked me. I blamed my husband.

I just kept saying: "You are to blame. You were not there when I needed you."

Inside I felt that I was wrong. I felt loneliness, helplessness, and fear. It had escalated rapidly in me, ruined my marriage, and corrupted my relationship with the world because of depression.

After two years I noticed that I no longer I saw myself for who I was, but I saw a complete stranger."

Another woman spelled out this period:

"I am a painter. At an exhibition opening a drunk man said that none of the pictures were really mine, I wasn't talented, what good is all this fuss for? Harsher and harsher words were due for my pictures.

The gallery staff removed him, but his words constantly rang in my head.

As if the devil would have repeated days later: "You're no good."

This incident crushed my self-confidence, I ruined my faith that I was a talented painter.

I locked myself in and did not paint any more.

Revenues froze, I did not sell more pictures.

Now I work in a factory as strip worker.

Then the man whom I did not know completely and permanently shielded my life."

We all live in different moments and periods of

"abduction".

However, what is common is the oblivion of the identity of the self.

The world which until then was the point of our lives is now cut seclusion.

Immersion is a moment that has become something of the past - it takes place shortly afterward.

However, it put me in this role, thereby limiting the happiness of my future.

Unlike the loss of personality, the awakening is very different, It takes many forms.

I feel that I met my three monsters of the underworld so that the awakening was third.

But none of them was the same as the others. The last realization of my personality abduction happened three years ago when a feeling of complete worthlessness gruelingly swirled in my soul.

My dreams of writing were shattered and I was unable to behold the sunny side of things.

The source of everyday niceties was meditation in my herb garden.

One day when I was sitting in my garden Teraxlation was born from the wonderful sentence:

"Embrace your heart with a loving hug."

For me, it was the awakening - the realization that I had not been myself lately.

As if the feelings of worthlessness scattered that small pieces of who I was. I looked around and everything reported pain - my surroundings, the people around me, my family, my financial situation. I lovingly embraced all my heart and accepted it.

Then I felt a complete whole and knew that the meditation had saved my life.

About Theresia

Theresia Valoczy is #1 Bestselling Author, Author of How To teach The Universal laws To Children International Best Selling Book, Certified in Indigo Studies, Hypnotherapist. Theresia coach female and young people to discover and find their passion, develop personality. Her main aim is to teach people how to use their creative energy and the Universal Laws, Angel Guidance to complete their Life.

www.spiritualparenting.eu

www.consciouscreatorspublishing.com

SET YOUR ALARM CLOCK

By Karen Wiltshire

Being awake in your life starts with self love. Letting go of thinking patterns, as well as behaviour patterns that block your true self from shining through. Replace those patterns with confidence, courage and grace to live an amazing unlimited life.

We are all responsible for our own happiness. Let Your heart, soul and mind be your compass . Life is chaotic at times and we forget to notice all the good that is right in front of us. Live with intention expect good things to come your way and they will. Focus on being grateful for what you have . Surround yourself with people and experiences that help you be the best you can be. Check in ith youself a fe tmes a day to measure your enegy. If your energy is positive then you will radiate a 'light' tht othr people want. You are in control of how you react to life. Choose peace and love ....what's the alternative?

Designing our own road map in this life can be somewhat trying, as we can grow up with counterfeit ideas of ourselves. These ideas so imprinted in our minds, that we believe them to be the truth. Thus making it way too easy to follow a path that is not our own - one that preoccupies and gets "in the way" of our true wants and desires.

As a woman coming into my own, it took great leaps of

faith and a cocktail of various struggles to discover and embrace this. There was a great lack of understanding on my part that yes, there is infact a spiritual plan for each and every one of us and we are never left alone.

I spent years in a state of despair and confusion. I know now after working on myself that I have a deep connection with the spiritual world, and I take comfort in the realization that this realm will always have my back. How many people are lucky enough to realize this? There is no doubt that my soul purpose will be fulfilled. It was not until I truly took the time to examine myself, that I felt the light switch on and I began to wake up. This light being only a faint flicker at first, served as a sign and helped me to let go of my jaded childhood beliefs and find my much deserved peace. My peace of power.

Everyone has their own struggles which become a part of their own unique story. Give yourself permission to not stay in that place that no longer serves you. Then, and only then, can you rewrite a more gentle ending to a story that started off toxic or tragic.

The overwhelming whirlwind of the highs and lows , wins and losses that presented themselves day in and day out throughout my lifetime, challenged me to be brave enough to fall and then get back up. I was strong enough to break. Now, I am very well aware that the power of my thoughts will continue to open pathways of acceptance, integrity, forgiveness, freedom, caring, encouragement, dedication, sharing, respect, gratitude, devotion, responsibility, energy, evolution, reliability, compassion, joy, cooperation, health, wellness, choice, chance , creativity, emotion all coming together into my very own dance.

There are times in our lives that we all come undone. Those dark whispers trying to claim a false version of ourselves. But guess what? It's ok to be human. Take these breakages into account and let them act as magnificant messages from heaven - as hidden treasures that are found in the broken pieces of ourselves. Redefining what a happy, successful life looks like requires discipline and time management, all the while being concious that these decisions that will be beneficial to my journey and therefore, that these decisions will be everlasting.

Untangling misguided beliefs of myself has allowed the stars to shine brighter, smells to be stronger, touch to be deeper, for new experiences to taste sweeter and sound to be harmonious . It is about the removal of that dark veil that suffocates your ideal self. Compare it to a caterpillar that spins a cocoon around itself for a season . Although it is dark, the caterpillar feels safe. As time passes the caterpillar know that he cannot stay in that state any longer, so with great expectancy for an abundant life the caterpillar starts to pump blood into its wings. Hopes and dreams can become a reality so the pumping continues. Then finally, at the appointed time, the wings break through and it takes flight. Find the strengh to break out of your own cocoon. Live with passion, gather the tools needed for further exploration to be your authentic self . Most importanly, release the expressions of those who hold no credentials for your life. It is time to set your alarm clock. Your abundant life is waiting for you.

"Sail on silver girl. Sail on by. Your time has come to shine. All your dreams are on their way, see how they shine. If you need a friend, I'm sailing right behind. Like a bridge over troubled water, I will ease your mind. Like a bridge over troubled water I will ease your mind." - Simon and Garfunkel

'Grief never ends...but it changes. It's a passage, not a place to stay. Grief is not sign of weakness or a lack of faith...it is a price for love'.

About Karen

Karen Wiltshire is a Transition Life Coach. She uses her intuitive sense, wisdom and knowledge to transition from one stage of life to the next. Whether it is a kiss of a loved one, separation or divorce, Karen brings courage and conviction to her clients.

www.yourpeaceofpower.com

HOW TO ENJOY YOUR MIDLIFE CRISIS

By Lira Kay

So you feel stuck and like nothing goes your way. You worry that the best years of your life are over. You look back and toss the memories, some exiting and some just plain care-free, and you wonder, will you ever have another chance to relive your past, to be as spirited and soulful as you once were.

I understand you completely. You are not alone. In every adult woman's and man's life there will be a turning point. It is not always defined by their age. But it just happens, that it is most likely to occur around us turning 40, or 50 if you are a man. Many report experiencing having the midlife crisis in their thirties, and some in their 60-s. The general feeling is a fear that life will never be the same again.

Many of my clients when I ask them what do they want to get out of coaching, say, "I just want my old self back". They tell me about their level of energy just a few years back, how busy and successful they were, how attractive and confident. They could take on the world. They could accomplish anything. They felt they have time. Now they feel tired, frustrated, often envious of they younger peers, like to complain and feel like they are constantly competing against time.

As the midlife crisis progresses what happens next is that they would make the last attempt to breakthrough and go for what they feel they are missing out on. They have the makeover, learn everything about the positive attitude, join social groups, start dating again, and try project kind of care-free attitude, they think, would separate them from the other mid-lifers. We've seen and, perhaps, experienced this phase ourselves. We would remember how highs would be replaced by the lows of dissatisfaction from feeling like a fraud. Fake it until you make it doesn't work, when you are a responsible mature adult. **You just can not replace what you feel inside by acting like you don't care**.

On the contrary, because we had reached midlife we have a chance to see life and ourselves for what it is. We have an urge to go deeper, look beyond surface. For us it is not just about showing others how well we did, but it's mainly about how well we feel about it.

Midlife is time of re-evaluation. Bit by bit we want to see the value in everything we've done over our life time. Often we feel regret for lost time, relationships and opportunities. Often we blame ourselves for not doing it right, for failing, for blowing it all together. More often than not we would justify all of that with circumstances. Life happened, we can all relate to that.

What is left for us to do? Our biggest fear is that life had stopped for us. Boring is the scariest word. No, we are not ready to be boring, balanced and peaceful. We still want to do and be something! But what can we be and what can we do? All we had been and done feels boring and overworked. It just doesn't have the same attraction.

Midlife crisis and identity crisis go hand in hand. Some times, and statists show that this is about 95% of us, actually, can not re-live what we had again. More than half of the marriages had ended, we accumulated a long list of things we have to take care of, including our own children, ailing parents, and many material possession. **Going back is not an option.**

So when you are experiencing your midlife crisis, the first thing is to see whether you are standing next to a beautiful house you want to continue living in, maintaining it and making some great additions. Or whether you are observing the ruins, that can be partly rebuilt. Or whether you are looking at the burned down to the bitter end house of which nothing can be saved. Is there a foundation left? Or this, too, needs to be put together brick by brick, perhaps, in the foreign land, that is more fertile and user friendly.

If you own the beautiful house, congratulations. You can stop reading this article. You are one of the lucky ones.

The rest of us can benefit from these three tips on how to enjoy your midlife crisis.

Tip number one: let yourself fully morn what you have lost and feel gratitude for what you have achieved.

This part is called: **validation**. When I begin working with a new client this the first thing we do. We don't miss taking account of anything, the good the bad and the ugly.

The tendency is usually focus on the losses and forget the gain. Because we tried to save the face, we had been posting inspirational quotes and some smily selfies on Facebook. The more we tried to keep our pain a secret, the more, when we had been left alone, we were caught up in self-criticism and negativity. Our psyche was balancing out the outer and inner inputs. So with validating yourself, you will bring that balance onto the surface, letting it empower you, instead of making you feel like you whole public life was a pretense.

Validation is a quiet process. What you know about yourself is for you only. As soon as you start sharing, you may fall into danger of telling a story, not the whole truth. The point of this exercise is to be truthful with yourself. One day, when time is right, and there will be any need for it, you can tell or write your story, make it an entraining read. But not yet. Let yourself really see your life and yourself in that life. Write about it in your own secret journal. It will do you a lot of good. Relief, gratitude, appreciation for your strength, is something to expect to feel after doing this exercise.

Tip number two: ask yourself, what have you learned?
One of the sad truths of life is that if we don't learn our life lessons we will keep repeating them over and over. I don't need to remind you about the strangest patterns, you notice, your life goes through. The only chance to get out of the vicious, or less than inspiring circle, is to find the nuggets of wisdom in your situation. What was that ex or that redundancy all about? What did you discover about yourself? **What do you know and own now because of that?**
Again, the best way to approach this exercise is to write a list of happenings in your life and then write the life lesson against each of them. You'll be surprised how wise you are. Also, feeling grateful for having been given a chance to learn and grow is not an uncommon feeling gained after this exercise.

Tip number three: Dare to dream!
I know, I know, it is scary. All your life you had been playing it half way, trying to protect yourself from criticism and disappointment. But here is another truth

about life: **you get what you ask for!** We are amazingly capable and also powerful beings. Once we know what we want our mind begins to do what it meant to do. Your mind will figure out how to get there the best way possible. I want to add some mystery to it and say, your life itself will figure it out and you will feel guided and supported on your quest. But you do need to have a quest. Dwelling on regrets is not something to look forward to in another decade or so. Why not do it? What is stopping you? How to overcome your blocks? All of those questions can be addressed after you established what is it you truly want from your life.

Now what else you would want to know about enjoying your midlife crisis, or better, your midlife transformation?

You don't have to do it alone. Like I mentioned, most of us had been there and done that, the hard way. It doesn't need to be the same for you. I know, that you had been searching for pain relief for some time already. You probably read every article and even done some on-line courses and such, to begin your midlife journey. But there's more to transformation then just reading the right books, or even hanging out with likeminded people. At some point you have to decide whether you are serious about living your life to the full. Are you ready to take yourself, your life seriously?

If your answer is yes, even if you have doubts whether you are worth it, or whether it is going to work, I invite you to get support. And not just any support, but a **professional support**. From somebody who is fully qualified and experienced in helping people to enjoy their midlife transformations. **Invest in yourself.**

With your happiness the life begins. The life that only you know. The only life you will ever know. The only journey you have to have, and the only path you have to walk. You are important. And the time is now or never.

I feel really passionate about this subject because I had seen my own parents live through their midlife crisis. They had no one to show them that crisis is a message from their own soul and spirit to step up and at last find yourself and be happy. From the age of 16 I started researching and learning about happiness, and looked for the ways to make the process of finding happiness a pleasant experience. After 20 plus years and many hundreds of people I had worked with I honed my skills as a life coach and feel confident I can take you there. I can show you **how your midlife crisis can become the best opportunity for growth and transformation.** You are worth it and I know it for sure.

You can find out more about my own midlife transformation journey on www.shesgotapssion.com ABOUT page.

About Lira

Lira Kay is international bestselling author, life coach specializing in dealing with self sabotage and fear of success, spiritual counselor and a founder of She's Got Passion and the School of Inspired Life a training center for purpose-driven professionals to find information and inspiration to stay on their mission to create a meaningful change in the world. Lira has been assisting people to transform their lives over twenty years, through art-therapy based workshops, practical seminars, transformative classes, psychotherapy, art, international curatorial projects—and now through coaching, speaking and spiritual healing sessions. After traveling the world, Lira settled in Walnut Creek, CA with her husband and their five daughters. Learn more at **www.LiraKay.com** and download Lira's free video training and PDF booklet, "Now or Never, How to Get What You Want Every Time You Say 'I Wish.'"

Book a free strategy session
http://www.shesgotpassion.com/get-acquainted-call

Get Free Video Course and a PDF copy of Lira's book

http://www.shesgotpassion.com/copy-of-now-or-never-free-video-tra

THE MAGICAL WORLD OF NUMBERS

JULY   ....   rest,   relax,   vacation

Even though the month of July starts out with picnics, fireworks and parades, this seventh month of the calendar year is just the opposite energetically. Chill out, kick back, go on vacations in July should become the norm. Statistically, more people go on vacation in July than any other month of the calendar year. Somehow the soul knows it needs to rest.

Physically, one can feel moopy-doopy under this seventh calendar month influence. "And God rested on the seventh day" certainly explains the sabbatical   energy   of   July.

As a transit in a personal chart during any given month, a *Seven says slow down your life*. If one does not slow down, their health can be used by the soul to just shut them down for many days with flu, colds, bodily injuries, disappointing relationships, financial woes that just need to be dealt   with.

As a personality, I call this birthday Number Seven the Greta Garbo energy...."I vant to be alone"!

Have you ever been to a party where all are displaying physical signs of hilarity and yet there is this one individual who seems to be "somewhere else"? Appearing unemotional, aloof, quiet and reserved, one gets the distinct impression he is viewing all emotionalism as rather immature.

If you have had this experience, you just might be in the presence of a person born on the seventh, sixteenth or twenty-fifth of any given month. Don't be misled, however. Beneath this analyzing, secretive energy breathes *a sensitive and caring individual.* Frequently, the emotions of the Number Seven are so buried in its spiritual and intuitive chemistry that they may never see the "light of day".

Finding spiritual connections in aloneness, this mystical and deep personality can drift off into philosophical dissertations that leave its listeners scratching their heads in wonderment.

The Number Seven is not one of the best financial energies so choices need to be made to keep monies in balance. The Number Seven temperament has the potential to be good in business but frequently does not follow through on its plans. On the other hand, there is a tendency to complete all projects in general.

The Number Seven is the ego Number causing an analytical and skeptical approach to life to be predominant. This then leads to a sense of perfectionism which in turn can cause difficulties in relationships. To be involved in a marriage with a Number Seven takes a special person who understands Number Seven's need to be alone. This is not the best basis for a fifty-fifty arrangement! The key is to *unlock the bottled-up emotions* that could create the rough times and once that is done and understood, Number Seven's personality tends to be a loyal and faithful marriage   partner.

Counteracting their fears and loneliness issues, Number Seven partners settle nicely into family life and greatly appreciate the affectionate gestures of loved ones. Number Seven energies tend to express love and feelings from a spiritual base and thus seem to have difficulty returning all the "hugs and kisses" in an effusive, emotional way.

When adding the month, day and year of birth together resulting in a Seven Number, know there will be a quest to discover truth within as the hallmark of this incarnation. However, the ego and mind are extremely powerful in this individual thus causing thinking and analyzing to *override the awesome intuitive and clairvoyant energy ability it possesses.*

The natural urge is to intellectually know and then to obtain specifics from a technical point of view all of life's experiences. The middle years of life from thirty to fifty-five, gently and intuitively nudges the human to develop a spiritual approach. It is this pushing by the soul that makes the personality want to be alone more. In the aloneness, the Higher Self can get through the ego and mind. Nature offers a very good support system by prompting the Number Seven to want to be in nature, around water, in the mountains or desert providing the solitude to just think.

At heart, Number Sevens love change and travel. *They have a very restless nature.* Their interest in far off lands often makes them extremely good writers, researchers, painters or poets. Interests also lie in computers, science or the occult. Whatever their interests, though, their own peculiar philosophy eventually creeps into their   work.

Number Sevens care little about the material things of life. If they become wealthy from their ideas or methods of business they are just as likely to make donations from their wealth to charities or institutions.

Although the Number Seven may say very little, he observes a great deal. His sense of dignity and the need for the finer things of life lead Number Seven to experience the joy of living. In an emergency situation, the Number Seven's first response is to pray.

This deeply introspective Number Seven energy, if off course, can be interpreted as "depression". To cover the hyper-intuitive rumblings going on within, Number Sevens may also turn to abuse of drugs and alcohol to quiet their inner selves down!

On a Sunday or Monday, the luck of Number Seven can intensify if various shades of green with white and yellow are worn. Moonstone, "cat-eye" or pearls round off the Number seven's lucky energy.

This quiet, introspective Number Seven personality brings to us all the gentle, spiritual vibrations that are so needed to slow us down in this fast-paced world we live in.

Number Sevens need to be a solitary figure, connecting the earth energy to all of us through it's intuitive and clairvoyant abilities. In doing so, it would justify it's reputation as the "Alone Ranger".

About Elizabeth

Spiritually guiding clients since 1988, Elizabeth Summers provides practical information by combining Numerology, Astrology and Tarot interpretations in her personal readings

For a private Numerology reading with Elizabeth Summers, please go here to review your choices: http://elizabethsummers.com/numerologyreadings.html

Website: www.elizabethsummers.com

Facebook: https://www.facebook.com/elizabeth.summers.338

You   Tube: https://www.youtube.com/channel/UCVPYhogOXHzJSXy UQFQuxLw

www.ingramcontent.com/pod-product-compliance
Lightning Source LLC
Chambersburg PA
CBHW071129280526
45787CB00003B/1221